YOUR KNOWLEDGE HAS VALUE

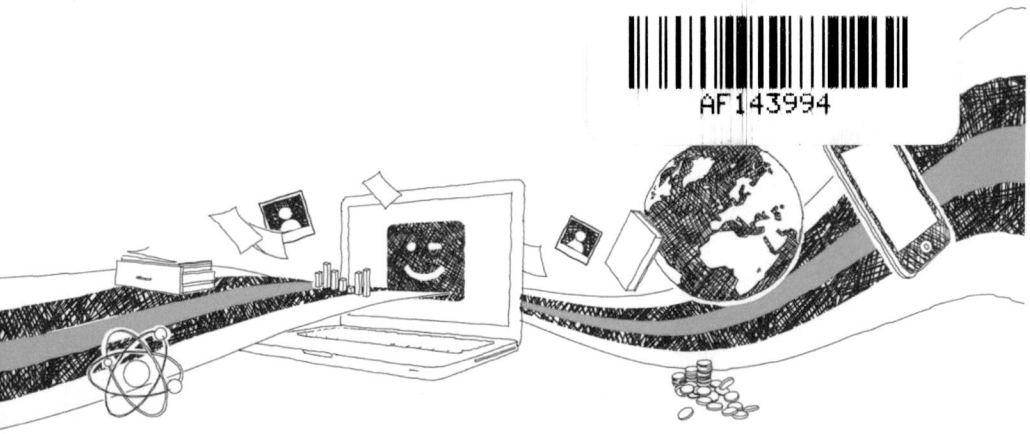
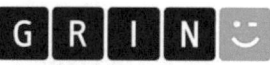

Bibliographic information published by the German National Library:

The German National Library lists this publication in the National Bibliography; detailed bibliographic data are available on the Internet at http://dnb.dnb.de .

Imprint:

Copyright © 2018 GRIN Verlag, Open Publishing GmbH
Print and binding: Books on Demand GmbH, Norderstedt Germany
ISBN: 9783668623170

This book at GRIN:

https://www.grin.com/document/388418

Patrick Kimuyu

The Comparative Effectiveness of Cytology Testing and HPV DNA Testing Based Primary Screening Pathways within a Cervical Screening Program

GRIN Publishing

GRIN - Your knowledge has value

Since its foundation in 1998, GRIN has specialized in publishing academic texts by students, college teachers and other academics as e-book and printed book. The website www.grin.com is an ideal platform for presenting term papers, final papers, scientific essays, dissertations and specialist books.

Visit us on the internet:

http://www.grin.com/

http://www.facebook.com/grincom

http://www.twitter.com/grin_com

The Comparative Effectiveness of Cytology Testing and HPV DNA Testing Based Primary
Screening Pathways within a Cervical Screening Program

Name: Patrick Kimuyu

Abstract

Primary screening of cervical cancer has been faced with an array of challenges which are attributable to the lack of appropriate technology. These challenges compromised the effectiveness of screening programs in different countries. It is apparent that the detection of cervical cancer precursors forms the basis for the success of screening programs for cervical cancer leading to the reduction of cervical cancer incidence and prevalence trends. Currently, there are two diagnostic methods that can be used for primary screening of cervical cancer: Pap cytology and HPV DNA test. However, the comparative effectiveness of this diagnostic tests indicate that HPV test is more effective than Pap cytology which is used as a first-line diagnostic method in cervical cancer prevention programs in many countries. Cytology testing and HPV testing differ significantly on the level of accuracy and sensitivity. Evidence studies indicate that HPV test exhibits high sensitivity and accuracy compared to Pap test. In a publicly-financed healthcare system such as the US, Canadian and EU, HPV testing has been proven to be more cost-effective than Pap test. Therefore, there is need to adopt HPV test for triage and primary screening.

Keywords: Pap cytology, HPV co-testing, human papillomavirus, sensitivity, first-line, negative, unclear, positive, colposcopy

Contents

Introduction.. 4

HPV Testing In Primary Cervical Cancer Screening 4

    HPV Testing in America 6

    HPV Testing in Canada.. 6

    HPV Testing in Australia 7

Cytology Testing In Primary Cervical Cancer Screening... 7

HPV Co-Testing (HPV + Cytology).. 8

Comparison between Cytology Testing and HPV DNA Testing 8

Sensitivity and Accuracy 8

    Cost-Effectiveness.. 9

    Vaccination Effect.. 10

Reason for Change of Primary Screening Strategy 10

    Factors Influencing Change of Strategy.. 10

Conclusion 10

References... 12

Introduction

Over the years, primary screening of cervical cancer has been faced with an array of challenges which are attributable to the lack of appropriate technology. These challenges compromised the effectiveness of screening programs in different countries. It is apparent that the detection of cervical cancer precursors forms the basis for the success of screening programs for cervical cancer leading to the reduction of cervical cancer incidence and prevalence trends. However, the introduction of new technology in screening for cervical cancer seems to have improved epidemiological responses through early detection of the disease. For instance, the application of human papillomavirus (HPV) DNA testing and cell (pap) cytology are currently considered the mainstay diagnostic pathways in primary screening for cervical cancer (1). However, these new technologies exhibit diverse degrees of effectiveness in the healthcare system. Therefore, this literature review focuses on the comparative effectiveness of HPV DNA testing and cytology testing based primary screening diagnostic methods within a cervical screening program.

HPV Testing In Primary Cervical Cancer Screening

HPV testing has been accepted as an alternative diagnostic method for primary screening of cervical cancer in women. This approach focuses on detecting HPV types that are believed to present a high risk of cervical cancer (2). HPV is a virus that infects the genital areas of humans. This virus is usually transmitted through sexual intercourse, and its infection does not manifest signs and symptoms (5). In most cases, the body fights off the infection by clearing the virus from the body through immune response mechanisms. Center for Disease Control and Prevention (CDC) reaffirms this phenomenon by stating HPV infection disappears within two years without causing any health problems, and this phenomenon is attributable to defense responses of the immune system (3). However, it has been found out that HVP causes cervical cancer after remaining in the cervical cells for a prolonged period. This occurs in two different ways depending on the type of HPV involved. Research indicates that some HPV types cause cervical cancer by causing changes on a woman's cervix. On the other hand, HPV can cause morphological changes in cervical cells; thus, leading to the development of genital warts (5). However, it is worth noting that the HPV types that have been found to be responsible for causing genital warts in both women and men are different from those that cause cervical cancer in women. Evidence studies indicate that genital HPVs comprises of more than 40 related HPV types which are responsible for most STIs. However, it is worth noting that only 14 HPV types are considered as significant etiological agents for cervical cancer. These are considered as 'high-risk' HPV types. Laine reports that often, a high-risk HPV infection is eliminated by the immune system and it does not manifest health problems. However, it is reported that 10% of women who are infected with high-risk HPV experience a persistent infection which increase the risk of cancer. Research indicates that HPV infections, primarily with 'high-risk' HPV types account for all cervical cancers. However, only two 'high-risk' HPV types cause about 70% of cervical cancers in women. Recent studies have identified HPV 16 and HPV 18 as the most virulent of all the genital HPVs (4).

Therefore, HPV DNA testing (HPV test) is meant for testing the presence of HPV types related to cervical cancer, but not all types. For instance, the cobas HPV test identifies the genome from the 'high-risk' HPV types. However, it exhibits specificity in the detection of HPV 16 and HPV 18, the most virulent 'high-risk' HPV types. Ordinarily, cervical cancer is common among women aged 30 years and beyond, although some cervical cancer cases have been reported in women at the ages of 20 and 29 years. Evidence studies indicate that HPV is not common in young women because they have an increased innate ability to fight off HPV infection within a few years compared to women older than 30 years (3). This is the reason HPV testing is recommended for screening of cervical cancer in women who are older than 30 years of age. It focuses on detecting HPV types which cause the growth of abnormal cervical cells or cervical cancer.

In practice, a negative HPV test implies the absence of any of the 'high-risk' HPV types in a woman; thus, the risk of cervical cancer is relatively low. On the other hand, a positive HPV test implies 'high-risk' HPV types are present. This implies that a woman is suffering or likely to suffer from cervical cancer (3). In the case of cobas HPV test, women with HPV 16 and HPV 18 are required to undergo colposcopy, in order to enable for the examination of cervical cells. As a result, it is possible to determine whether a woman who tests positive for the two HPV types has abnormal cervical cells, a characteristic of cervical cancer, or it has not yet set. On the other hand, a positive test for the other 12 high-risk HPV types does not warrant for colposcopy. In this case, a Pap test is performed to determine the necessity of colposcopy (4). However, the application of HPV test depends on the guidelines stipulated by different countries.

HPV Testing in America

In the United States, HPV testing was first approved in 2011 for use as a follow-up to cell cytology. This was followed by a three-year's clinical study which involved 40,000 women older than 25 years of age. Women who screened positive for HPV or showed positive Pap test underwent a cervical tissue biopsy and colposcopy and all the results were compared, in order to ascertain the safety and effectiveness of HPV testing. It was from the results of this study that FDA approved HPV test as a new option for primary cervical cancer screening, in April 2014. The approval of HPV test expanded the application of the test; it can be used for primary screening or co-testing (4). This is expected to enhance the success of cervical cancer screening programs in the US. Currently, epidemiological reports indicate that more than 16 out of every 100,000 women in the US, aged 40 years and older develop cervical cancer each year (3).

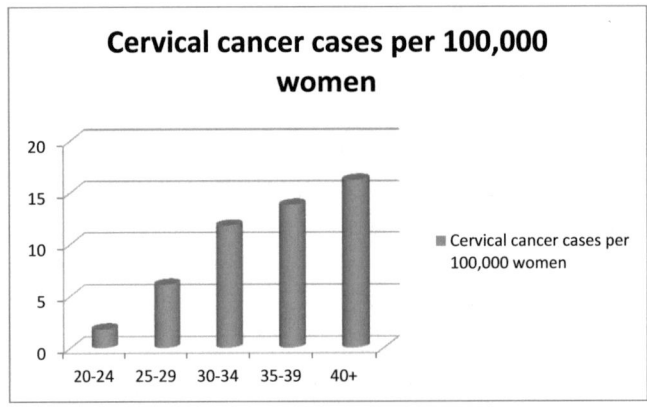

HPV Testing in Canada

In Canada, HPV test is approved for use in women, although its application in cervical cancer screening is limited. Public Health Agency of Canada reports that HPV DNA testing does not serve as screening tests or a Pap test; instead, it is recommended for certain situations. This is so because Pap test is considered the gold standard for primary screening of cervical cancer. Therefore, HPV test is a follow-up test to determine the need for repeat cytology and management (5).

HPV Testing in Australia

Australia has been using Pap cytology for primary screening in cervical cancer programs. As such, HPV DNA testing is not considered as a first-line diagnostic approach for cervical cancer screening (14). However, HPV test is used for the management of cervical cancer in women treated for a high-grade abnormality. In this case, HPV test is not performed for screening purposes, but rather for therapeutic purposes, especially determining the elimination of HPV virus from the body after treatment (6).

Cytology Testing In Primary Cervical Cancer Screening

Cytology screening has been considered as the traditional primary diagnostic method for cervical cancer careening in women. Sorbye et al admit the differences in the effectiveness of these triage methods by stating HPV triage is more sensitive than cytology (11). Ordinarily, Pap cytology focuses on the development of abnormal cervical cells which can grow into cervical cancer. This test is ideal for women who are older than 21 years, and it has been considered a gold standard for cervical cancer screening programs in many countries. According to CDC, Pap test produces three results: normal (negative), unclear or abnormal based on the morphology of cervical cells. Normal Pap test results imply that a woman's cervical cells do not show changes; thus, there is no risk of cervical cancer. However, this does not mean that a woman will not develop cervical cancer in the future. As a result, women who test negative for Pap test are required to go for screening after three years because new cell changes can occur in the cervix. On the other hand, unclear Pap test results imply that a woman's cervical cells reveal abnormal changes which are not specific for HPV. Evidence studies indicate that cell changes in the cervix are attributable to life changes including menopause, pregnancy or infection, primarily HPV. Finally, an abnormal Pap test results indicate that cervical cells manifest changes. This suggests that HPV may be responsible for the observed cell changes. However, this does not mean that a woman with abnormal Pap test results has cervical cancer. Cell changes are either low-grade (minor) or high-grade (serious). High-grade cell changes are commonly referred to as 'pre-cancer' because they can advance into cancer over time (6).

HPV Co-Testing (HPV + Cytology)

The use of HPV test and cytology test concurrently has been found to be effective in early detection of cervical cancer in women. This is so because the sensitivity of Pap cytology varies from that of HPV testing. In the US, both cytology test and HPV test are used in primary screening. It is at the discretion of physicians and the preference of patients to choose either Pap test or HPV test for cervical cancer screening. It is reported that the HPV-Pap strategy in a cervical cancer screening program decreases the risk of cancer by 78-93% compared to 81-90% rate reported for Pap test alone (12). However, the situation is relatively different in Canada and Australia where Pap test is considered the first-line diagnostic in cervical cancer screening programs. This is probably attributable to the success realized through the adoption of Pap cytology in high-income countries. It is reported that in high-income countries, population-wide, cytology based screening has reduced mortality rates for cervical cancer (9). In these countries, HPV testing is used for follow-up purposes, but not for screening.

Comparison between Cytology Testing and HPV DNA Testing

Sensitivity and Accuracy

It is evident that HPV testing differs from cytology testing in an array of factors such as cost-effectiveness, interval, age, and vaccination effect. Foremost, cytology testing and HPV testing differ significantly on the level of accuracy and sensitivity. Evidence studies indicate that HPV test exhibits high sensitivity and accuracy compared to Pap test. Chow and his colleagues reaffirm that HPV DNA testing is more sensitive and accurate compared to Pap test (12). This aspect has been reaffirmed by other studies. For instance, Sorbye et al state that HPV tests can be used to locate lesions which cannot be identified through the use of cytology testing; thus, it is believed to increase clinical sensitivity of screening programs (11). According to Roche, the adoption of HPV DNA testing as first-line screening diagnostic leads to the identification of cervical cancer at a higher rate than using cytology testing alone. This implies that the high sensitivity associated with HPV testing enhances its accuracy. In some situations, Pap test shows abnormalities; thus, creating the need for HPV testing for confirmatory purposes. In contrast, HPV testing detects high-risk HPV types; thus, there is no need for confirmatory clinical tests.

8

Cost-Effectiveness

Secondly, these two diagnostic strategies manifest differences in cost-effectiveness. In general, screening has been found to be a significant cost-effective approach in preventing cervical cancer. It is apparent that all countries with cervical cancer screening have realized a significant reduction in cervical cancer related health consequences. As a result, the disease burden of cervical cancer is usually reduced compared to the situation where primary screening strategies are absent. In a publicly-financed healthcare system such as the US, Canadian and EU, HPV testing appears to be more cost-effective than Pap test. Evidence indicates that HPV testing has proven to be ideal for improving health effectiveness in developed countries compared to Pap test (12). This aspect is attributable to several factors. First, the intervals of screening for both HPV test and Pap test are variable with Pap test having a shorter screening interval than HPV test. In countries where Pap cytology is used as the first-line screening method for cervical cancer, the recommended interval is one year. This implies that women are required to go for Pap test, annually. As a result, the annual visits to physicians increase the cost of screening. In contrast, HPV test interval ranges from 3 to 5 years. This implies that women under HPV triage have few visits to physicians compared to those enrolled under cytology triage. On the other hand, HPV testing appears more cost-effective than cytology on the basis of the overall cost of treatment. Ordinarily, Pap test is ideal for women who are older than 21 years of age. In contrast, HPV test is ideal for use in women who are older than 30 years of age. However, the test can be performed in women aged 18 years, the age when most women become sexually active. The rationale for recommending HPV test at the age of 30 years is based on the fact that young women exhibit the ability to fight off HPV infections (3). Evidence shows that high-risk HPV types are likely to cause cervical cancer in older women than young ones, especially those who are below 30 years.

Therefore, commencing Pap screening at the age of 21 years, when there are few chances of high-risk HPV infections increases medical costs. Evidence indicates that the positive predictive value (PPV) of HPV test does not depend on cytology but rather the age of the women tested (10). In addition, Pap tests which turn out unclear require repeat cytology for the confirmation of HPV infection. As a result, repeat cytology increases the cost of screening under cytology triage in primary screening cervical cancer programs. It is also reported that Pap test is associated with a high number of referral for colposcopy compared to HPV testing.

9

Vaccination Effect

Moreover, cytology and HPV testing exhibit differences in vaccination effect. Evidence studies indicate that vaccination against HPV virus is associated with increased potential for the prevention of cervical cancer compared to Pap screening. This is so because protection from vaccination has been proven to last for at least 5 years. As a result, both direct and indirect medical costs are reduced through reducing Pap cytology and colposcopy. On the other hand, Pap testing is not age-specific compared to HPV testing. Therefore, HPV triage in young women and primary screening in older women appears consistent with vaccination (8).

Reason for Change of Primary Screening Strategy

In general, the comparative effectiveness of cytology testing and HPV testing based primary screening in cervical cancer screening program suggests that HPV test is effective for both triage in young women and primary screening in older women. Therefore, it is necessary for the adoption of HPV test as first-line diagnostic strategy for prevention of cervical cancer. The increased sensitivity, cost-effectiveness and reliability in cervical cancer vaccination presents the benefits associated with HPV testing which are far beyond the benefits associated with Pap cytology.

Factors Influencing Change of Strategy

In most cases, changes of disease prevention strategies are influenced by the cost of the strategy, reproducibility including sensitivity and accuracy of the primary diagnostics and policy regulations by international agencies such as the World Health Organization. Ordinarily, primary screening requires cost-effective diagnostic methods coupled with accuracy.

Conclusion

Cancer screening programs in different countries have been faced with challenges; thus, compromising their success. As a result, the epidemiological trends of cervical cancer seem to have remained unchanged despite the efforts made in early detection of the disease. However, the discovery of new diagnostic methods such as cobas HPV DNA testing appears to promote prevention strategies in different countries. It is apparent that screening plays significant roles in reversing the epidemiological trends of all diseases, and this has been the case with cervical cancer. Evidence shows that cervical cancer screening in women has reduced the morbidity and mortality associated with cervical cancer, worldwide.

In primary screening for cervical cancer, Pap cytology which looks for changes in the cervical cells has been the traditional method of detecting cervical cancer for early intervention. However, the discovery of molecular markers such as HPV DNA test has introduced an alternative diagnostic for primary screening. It is comparative that HPV test is highly effective compared to the traditional cytology testing. Therefore, the effectiveness of HPV test justifies its adoption for both triage and primary screening in cervical cancer programs.

References

1. Saslow D. et al. American Cancer Society, American Society for Colposcopy and Cervical Pathology, and American Society for Clinical Pathology screening guidelines for the prevention and early detection of cervical cancer. CA: A Cancer Journal for Clinicians. 2012 May-Jun; 62(3): 147–172.

2. Pileqqi C, Flotta D, Bianco A, Nobile C, Pavia M. Is HPV DNA testing specificity comparable to that of cytological testing in primary cervical cancer screening? Results of a meta-analysis of randomized controlled trials. Int J Cancer. 2014 Jul; 135(1):166-77.

3. CDC. Cervical cancer screening with the HPV test and the Pap test in women ages 30 and older [Internet]. [Cited 2014 Aug 20]. Available from http://www.cdc.gov/cancer/hpv/pdf/HPV_Testing_2012_English.pdf

4. Laine S. FDA approves first human papillomavirus test for primary cervical cancer screening [Internet]. [Cited 2014 Aug 20]. Available from http://www.cdc.gov/cancer/hpv/pdf/HPV_Testing_2012_English.pdf

5. Public Health Agency of Canada. What everyone should know about human papillomavirus (HPV): questions and answers [Internet]. [updated 2012 Oct 9; cited 2014 Aug 20]. Available from http://www.phac-aspc.gc.ca/std-mts/hpv-vph/pdf/hpv-vph-qa-eng.pdf

6. Australian Government. National cervical screening program: HPV (human papillomavirus) [Internet]. [updated 2012 Oct 9; cited 2011 May 14]. Available from http://www.cancerscreening.gov.au/internet/screening/publishing.nsf/Content/hpv

7. Phillips C. HPV and Pap co-testing safely extend cervical cancer screening intervals. National Cancer Institute. 2011 May; 8(11): 4.

8. Goldhaber-Fiebert, J. et al. Cost-Effectiveness of cervical cancer screening with human papillomavirus DNA testing and HPV-16, 18 vaccination. J Natl Cancer Inst. 2011 May; 100(5): 308–320.

9. Bosgraaf R. et al. Triage by methylation-marker testing versus cytology in women who test HPV-positive on self-collected cervicovaginal specimens (PROHTECT-3): a randomised controlled non-inferiority trial. Lancet Oncol. 2014; 15: 315–22.

10. Kelly R, Patnick J, Kitchener H, Moss, S. HPV testing as a triage for borderline or mild dyskaryosis on cervical cytology: results from the Sentinel Sites study. British Journal of Cancer. 2011; 105: 983 – 988.

11. Sørbye S. et al. Triage of Women with Low-Grade Cervical Lesions - HPV mRNA Testing versus Repeat Cytology. PLoS ONE. 2011 Aug; 6(8): e24083.

12. Chow I. et al. Cost-effectiveness analysis of human papillomavirus DNA testing and Pap smear for cervical cancer screening in a publicly financed health-care system. British Journal of Cancer. 2010; 103: 1773 – 1782.

13. Techakehakij W, Feldman R. Cost-effectiveness of HPV vaccination compared with Pap smear screening on a national scale: A literature review. Vaccine. 2008; 26: 6258–6265.

14. Boone D, Erickson B, Huh W. "New insights into cervical cancer screening", Journal of Gynecologic Oncology, 2012; 23(4):282-287.

YOUR KNOWLEDGE HAS VALUE

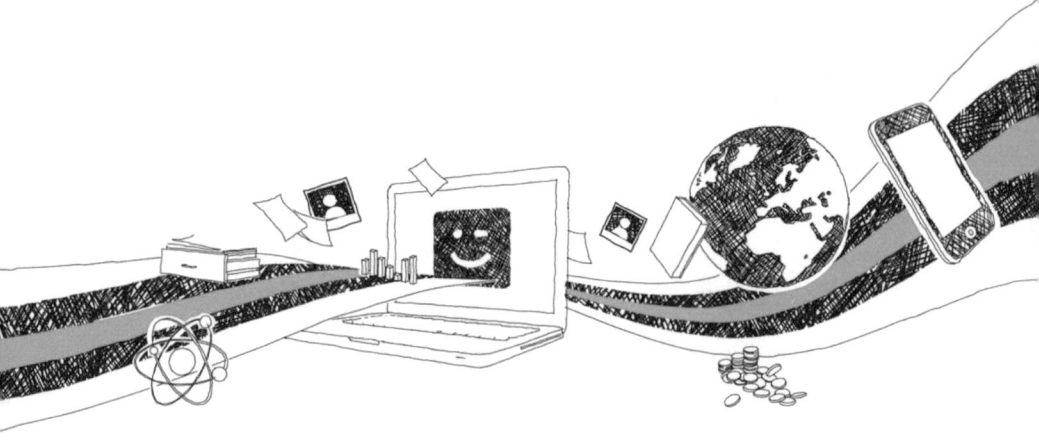

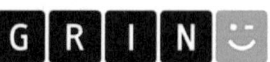